Blood Pressure Tracker

Date	Systolic	Diastolic	Heart Rate	Remarks

Blood Pressure Tracker

Date	Systolic	Diastolic	Heart Rate	Remarks

Blood Pressure Tracker

Date	Systolic	Diastolic	Heart Rate	Remarks

Blood Pressure Tracker

Date	Systolic	Diastolic	Heart Rate	Remarks

Blood Pressure Tracker

Date	Systolic	Diastolic	Heart Rate	Remarks

Blood Pressure Tracker

Date	Systolic	Diastolic	Heart Rate	Remarks

Blood Pressure Tracker

Date	Systolic	Diastolic	Heart Rate	Remarks

Blood Pressure Tracker

Date	Systolic	Diastolic	Heart Rate	Remarks

Blood Pressure Tracker

Date	Systolic	Diastolic	Heart Rate	Remarks

Blood Pressure Tracker

Date	Systolic	Diastolic	Heart Rate	Remarks

Blood Pressure Tracker

Date	Systolic	Diastolic	Heart Rate	Remarks

Blood Pressure Tracker

Date	Systolic	Diastolic	Heart Rate	Remarks

Blood Pressure Tracker

Date	Systolic	Diastolic	Heart Rate	Remarks

Blood Pressure Tracker

Date	Systolic	Diastolic	Heart Rate	Remarks

Blood Pressure Tracker

Date	Systolic	Diastolic	Heart Rate	Remarks

Blood Pressure Tracker

Date	Systolic	Diastolic	Heart Rate	Remarks

Blood Pressure Tracker

Date	Systolic	Diastolic	Heart Rate	Remarks

Blood Pressure Tracker

Date	Systolic	Diastolic	Heart Rate	Remarks

Blood Pressure Tracker

Date	Systolic	Diastolic	Heart Rate	Remarks

Blood Pressure Tracker

Date	Systolic	Diastolic	Heart Rate	Remarks

Blood Pressure Tracker

Date	Systolic	Diastolic	Heart Rate	Remarks

Blood Pressure Tracker

Date	Systolic	Diastolic	Heart Rate	Remarks

Blood Pressure Tracker

Date	Systolic	Diastolic	Heart Rate	Remarks

Blood Pressure Tracker

Date	Systolic	Diastolic	Heart Rate	Remarks

Blood Pressure Tracker

Date	Systolic	Diastolic	Heart Rate	Remarks

www.ingramcontent.com/pod-product-compliance
Lightning Source LLC
Chambersburg PA
CBHW051953280526
45789CB00009B/3273